In My Mind

My Journey to Hope

by Rowena Bernal

First Edition

ISBN: 978-621-96335-3-6

Published by:

Alphabet House Book Publishing
Malabanban Sur, Candelaria, Quezon
Contact Number: 09175551871
Email: alhousepublishing@gmail.com

This book is dedicated to you who continue to hope, nourish the hope in your heart, and give hope to others despite all the struggles and difficulties.

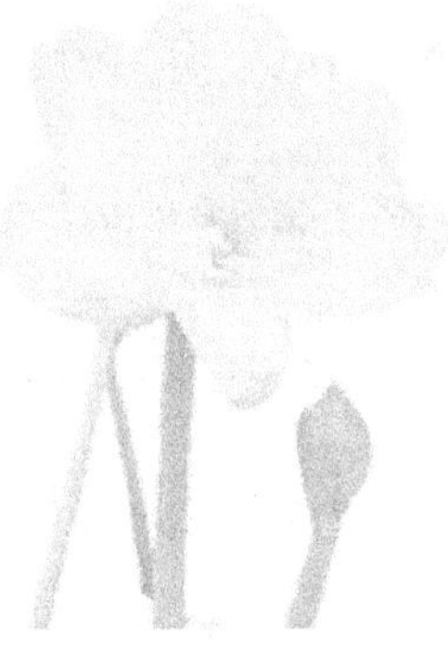

Disclaimer

This book is a work of fiction. The names, description of characters, places, events and incidents are the products of the author's imagination. Any resemblance to actual persons, living or dead, or actual events is purely coincidental and unintentional.

You are strong.

You are wonderful.

You have amazing gifts.

You have flaws.

You make mistakes.

You are not perfect.

You are special.

You are loved.

This is all of you.

I care for you. I wish the best for you.

I pray that blessings be showered upon you.

Happy Reading!

Introduction

A day consists of 24 hours, where a few hours are dedicated to sleep so that the body and mind can rest and recharge. Unless you are from a different universe or galaxy, or, if you are like me, your mind can make your day feel like a week, a month or a year. In 24 hours, your mind might be battling a thousand problems and coping with a hundred things all at the same time, and the emotional and mental toll can be so much more. Way, way more.

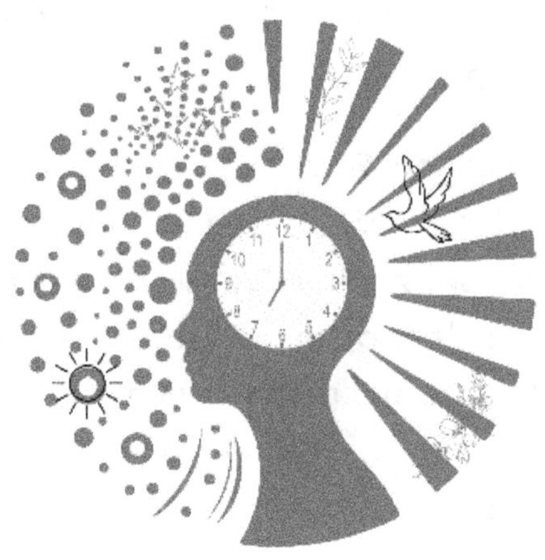

My grandmother used to say, "start the day right."

Bzzzzzz.....Bzzzz....."

The buzzing sound from my cellphone was so loud it filled my room and shook my eardrums. I thought I was in a nightmare where bees took over and I was the only human being who survived. It took some time for me to realize that it was my cellphone's alarm clock. I tried to ignore it but its incessant buzzing permeated every part of my brain so I decided I did not have a choice but to wake up.

"No!!!!! Stay in bed. Go back to sleep." A voice in my head ordered me. I wanted to follow that voice but I knew I shouldn't. In slow motion, I raised my eyelids to open my eyes. My left eyelid nicely cooperated and partially went up. My right eyelid, unfortunately, disagreed and remained closed. I was going to close my left eye again when the buzzing sound came back.

"Ahhh....I should have set the snooze for an hour!" Snooze is what I love and hate with alarms – it helps you wake up, I mean really wake up, but it is also annoying, especially when you want to go back to sleep.

I opened both eyes, raised my arms above my head, and yawned with my mouth wide open while my mid torso rose up a little bit as my head pressed harder on my soft, fluffy pillow. As soon as my yawn ended and my body settled back in bed, I felt a sense of dread settle over me. I cannot fully explain it but it was as if a cold, dark, threatening set of clouds got inside my room – although all windows were closed – and completely wrapped my body. I felt something heavy and cold in my heart, in my hands, and in my skin but that "something" was invisible and indescribable. I shivered at the cold and the confusion.

Suddenly, my whole body felt tired. I had just woken up but I felt spent and devoid of energy. How do you start your day with these draining and depressing emotions?

"I don't want to get up. I don't want to go to work. Oh my God! Work. I can't work. I don't want to work." I knew that once my day started with this tug-of-war in my head, it's going to be a bad day. Not a whole day bad day kind but a complicated, emotionally draining kind of bad day.

"Oh, I have a meeting. I need to go to work." I moaned.

The back and forth in my head was so overwhelming and made me feel like I was in limbo with one side ready to get up and the other pulling myself back to bed. My eyes were starting to get moist and tears were threatening to flow. It was a very difficult decision to make.

"I really don't want to go to work. What's the point of going to work? Why do I have to go to work? Who are the people I don't want to see? Well…none, they are all nice." Even my internal discussion with myself was confusing.

"Yeah, they are all nice. Maybe seeing them will make my day better." I smiled to myself.

"No, I don't want to see any of them. I don't want to see all of them. Mary, the receptionist will be smiling. Terry, my boss will be smiling. No! I don't want to see them smile. What in hell will they be smiling about? Oh, God, smiles annoy me." Another voice in my head contradicted my earlier thought.

I put my hands up to cover my face and then pulled my hair backward.

"Oh God, please don't let this be one of those days. Please, please, please. I don't have the energy right now. I am spent. Last week was horrible. It's too soon for another one of those days. Please, please, please dear God, don't let this day be one of those days."

I sat up and slid my legs down from my bed. I raised my head in a prayer-like move, hoping heaven was really in that direction, hoping that God was listening, and hoping that my prayer would be granted.

"No, no, no, please no."

I kept repeating it in my head while my hands were tapping my knees and, synching with the hands, my feet tapping the floor. It was as if the tapping of my hands was fueling the movement of my knees and feet. Then, I fell back on my bed with my eyes open, my mind blank, and with an overall feeling of fatigue and malaise.

It was a painful start.

"I need to take a shower. Yeah, that's what I need." I was pretty sure the shower would make things better because it would help awaken my senses and all I needed to feel better was to be fully awake. I raised my arms over my head, put my palms together, and yawned with full force, opening my mouth as wide as I could and letting out an incredibly loud yawning sound.

I stood up, walked purposefully towards the shower, finding my goal for waking up at last. As the water from the shower splashed on my face, it dawned on me that I had always been alone. Even when I was with my family, I was alone. Even when I was with my boyfriend, I was alone. Even when I was with friends, I was alone. Even when I was surrounded by people, I was alone. No one truly understood me. No one knew how I felt.

I remembered very clearly the first time I really felt so alone and insignificant. It was many years ago. I was by myself in the apartment I was sharing with three other friends. It was right after work. As soon as I arrived at the apartment, I received a call from home. There were some problems again. I could not recall the problems anymore, but I remembered feeling spent and totally devoid of strength and energy when the call ended.

I sat on the floor helplessly. Both my hands were on my lap, with open palms facing upward, my right hand still had my phone but I was not holding it anymore. It was just sitting on my open right palm because I did not have the slightest strength needed to close my fingers around my phone. My head was bent so low you'd think it would eventually fall off from my neck. I was crying and my chest felt like it was drowning and was ready to explode.

I let out a painful, loud wail while releasing all the heaviness in my chest. I asked God why nothing was ever enough in my life. I asked God why I felt so tired. I asked God so many things. I blamed God for feeling alone, scared, helpless, and trapped. I was angry with him. I told him he was not real and I didn't believe in him. I told him that if he's real, he would have understood my pain and my life and he would have made things better. I confronted him.

"Didn't you say, come to me those who are tired and heavily laden and I will give you rest? Well, I am tired. My shoulders cannot carry my cross anymore, why won't you help me?"

I kept on crying for some time until my tears ran out and even the energy to cry had run its course. I slowly stood up and walked to the kitchen to get some water. Before I could get some water, I sat on the kitchen stool, closed my eyes, and did the only thing that I could do – I prayed. No matter how angry I was with God, there was really nothing else that I could hold on to at that point.

It was really ironic. You see, my prayers remained my sanctuary, yet, at that point, I could not feel God's presence anymore and I could not feel his helping hand. But I derived comfort from the knowledge that while I had no one in this world to be with me, to listen to me, and to comfort me, there was an unseen, all-knowing entity that sees me and knows me and all my pain and sufferings. Even when I doubted God, I hoped he was real. And even if he was not, the idea that he existed and that I could talk to him calmed me. Just the idea of God, more than anything else, kept me going.

"Damn! Why did I let myself think about it. I know what's going to happen next and I have no control over it." I scolded myself.

I started crying with my tears mixing with water from the shower. A muffled cry came out of my mouth. I covered my mouth with one hand to stop myself from crying while my other hand held onto the wall for support. It was no use. I couldn't stop crying. Maybe if I cry as hard as I can, this will be over soon.

"You need to cry. Let it out." There was someone in my mind. I was aware of the voices in my head and I felt like it was not me but someone else.

In a way, it was funny because the scene was like that TV commercial for a bath soap where the mother's conscience was advising her what kind of bath soap to use for the family. It started out as one voice and then became like a chorus. The more voices I heard in my head, the louder I cried, and the lonelier I felt.

"No, this life is not worth living."

"It's pointless."

"It's useless."

"It's painful."

All these voices were crowding inside my head. They were all screaming for space and attention. But all I wanted was for them to go away. I did not want what the voices made me feel. I started pulling my hair. I was not sure whether I was pulling my hair because the voices might go away as I yank my hair or because the pain from pulling my hair would make me forget about the voices.

When pulling my hair failed, I started banging my head on the wall while shouting, "Leave me alone! Go away! All of you, leave my head alone!" When the pain was enough to drown the voices in my head, I stopped. I held my tender, swollen head and silently cried, resting my back on the wall for support.

With immense struggle and determination, I managed to finish my shower. I splashed my eyes with cold water repeatedly to help lessen the puffiness of my eyes from too much crying. I got dressed and ate my breakfast. I moved fast as I did not want to be late for work. I had so many things to do.

Enjoy the little things.

I took one long look at my apartment as I was standing at the door, making sure I did not forget to turn off any electrical items or leave anything I needed. I locked the doorknob and turned the key for the double lock. I put the key in the inside pocket of my tote back, turned around, and started walking really fast.

"Hi, Annie! Good morning."

"Jackie! Hi! I didn't know you're back. How was your vacation?" I asked my neighbor, my eyes sparkling with happiness at seeing my neighbor back from her vacation. Suddenly, I was full of energy and enthusiasm.

"Just yesterday afternoon. Hey, drop by the house when you get off work. I brought something for you." Jackie looked excited.

"Wow! Thank you. I will sure drop by." I walked away still smiling. She's such a sweet neighbor. I raised my head sideways and squinted my eyes to take a look at the rays of the sun passing through the soft, veil-like clouds, which I think were called cirrus clouds.

"This is such a beautiful day and I am the luckiest person in the whole wide world. Why did I ever feel sad this morning?" I asked myself with a smile.

My forehead wrinkled as I tried to recall the heavy feelings I had this morning and to my amazement and bewilderment, I couldn't feel even the slightest sadness or anger in my heart. Instead, it was bursting with happiness, gratitude, and excitement for what lies ahead. There was so much happiness in my heart that I just knew for sure that things were going to be better. I took a deep breath. As the air reached the top of my nostrils, and my head slightly moved back, I closed my eyes, held the air for a few seconds, and released it while opening my eyes, taking in the mesmerizing view of a new morning, a new beginning.

This was the kind of morning that I like - warm but not hot. The sunshine was just enough to make me feel nice and the wind was blowing softly so my hair moved a little bit too. I liked the slight movement of my hair touching my face. I liked how stray strands of my hair went in front of my face and I had to brush them with my hand to the side or put them behind my ear. I felt so beautiful while I did that. I caught myself doing exactly that and I smiled. "Silly me."

I like watching people and today was no different. I once had a Sociology class where we were required to observe people in a mall. We were to observe them and try to figure out how their day went or who they were or their background by watching their movement and their interactions with people around them. I enjoyed that activity. I sat in the farthest corner of a mall food court, facing the entrance. I watched the people coming in. Even when there were many people coming in at the same time, one would always stand out. I didn't know why or how but someone would always draw my attention away from the rest. It was very interesting how that activity helped me understand people better. It also helped me think and act kinder towards others.

I realized that while walking, I was doing the same activity.

"Of all the people walking in this street today, is there anyone who has the same struggles as me? Is there anyone whose background is the same as mine? Isn't it amazing that, even though there are billions of people in this world, my story, my life is totally unique and special?"

When I thought about it, I felt really special and insignificant both at the same time. I felt special because I was the only one in this world with the combination of everything that made me "ME." But I also felt insignificant because no matter how big my personal problems were, I was but a speck of dust in this infinite universe.

"I need to appreciate life more, be more grateful, and just live for the moment. Life is beautiful, it is always beautiful. I just need to stop and live in the moment to enjoy it." I reminded myself.

As I continued walking, I saw a big, beautiful, yellow hibiscus starting to bloom. I stopped walking and stepped closer to look at the flower. As I did, I noticed a partly destroyed leaf with a caterpillar underneath. I watched the caterpillar. I could have been a biologist and I would be studying all living things.

I smiled. I remembered that time in grade school when my teacher asked me what I wanted to be when I grew up. I said I wanted to be a caterpillar because I wanted to become a beautiful butterfly and have wings so colorful, beautiful, and powerful, and be friends with the flowers. My teacher really loved my answer, and I know for sure I became her favorite student from that moment on.

"Oh, if only I really am the caterpillar right now." I sighed and imagined the splendid butterfly that would become of me, the caterpillar.

With my head full of happy thoughts and my heart filled with joy, I kept walking. Then, a thought popped into my mind. It was me going to work. I was a successful, kind, humble, and charismatic leader of a large organization. I was walking from my office to my apartment. I walked every day even though I had a very, very nice, sleek, and expensive car because walking made me one with the rest of my staff. While walking, I saw a woman who looked hungry and fragile, smelled really bad, and was being bullied by passersby. I walked over to the woman and became her champion.

"Is everything okay, Ma'am?" I asked her.

She looked at me and said, "Yes, I'm okay. I know I smell bad but there's nothing I can do to change that right now." I looked at her and saw how shrunken her face was like she had not eaten for days!

"Oh no!" I muttered as I felt myself slowly slipping into the make-believe world in my mind. I tried to stay in the present. I looked around me and tried to focus on one thing in my surroundings but the story in my mind was so overwhelming and so real.

The story in my head continued. I looked at her closely and saw the disappointment, frustration, and pain in her eyes. She was homeless and no matter how much she would have liked to look better and smell better, her current circumstances did not make that possible. I extended my hand and offered a handshake.

I said, "It's a privilege to meet you, Ma'am. I am so sorry that his world has been horrible to you. Please take this money. This will help you get by for a few days. Find a good place to stay for a week, rest, eat well, and take good care of yourself." She took the money with tears in her eyes. Everyone around us had their heads bowed knowing in their hearts that they had been amiss in their duty as human beings to help those in need.

I smiled and stopped walking. I was disoriented. I temporarily lost track of everything around me. The story was finished but another thought was taking shape.

"Oh, this darn head is taking me somewhere else again. Focus, Focus, Focus! You're going to work. Stop daydreaming!" I ordered my mind.

I shook my head really hard and focused on the "moment." A friend gave me a book about being focused. There was a tip on what can help you stay focused and remain in the "NOW" moment. It said you should listen intently to the sounds around you and identify them. Then, focus on one sound. I did that. I focused on the sound of passing cars.

Then, I remembered this one time when I was a college student. I was walking home with a friend and my mind started working on its own. I can't remember what I was thinking about anymore, but my friend shook my shoulders and said, "Why were you so angry while looking at the rocks? You scared me." I looked at her in confusion and realized that my anger at the situation in my mind was visibly shown on my face.

I had come to realize that my mind was my sanctuary but it had become scary too. It had been more active lately, like it had a mind of its own, which was ironic because it's my mind. MINE. When I felt embarrassed, shy or scared, I created an alternate reality in my mind where I controlled the events and the entire narrative. It had become so habitual and a part of my life that sometimes, I would read an email, craft a reply in my mind, and be so satisfied with that reply that I would forget or put off replying in real life. It was scary.

There were times when the story in my head became so powerful that I was physically immobilized. Whatever I was doing or where ever I was, I would stop to let the story in my head have a satisfying conclusion.

For example, I was washing the dishes and a story popped into my mind. What I did was I stopped washing the dishes, closed my eyes, and allowed my head to finish the story. It was like watching an interactive movie. Events were happening but I can change some of them. Another time, I was seated on the sofa, watching TV when a conversation in my mind overtook what I was watching. I stopped watching, stared in the distance, and continued the conversation in my head.

There was also a time when I was in bed and was about to sleep when a story came up in my head. I delayed going to sleep to finish the story in my head. My mind refused to do anything else until the story or conversation in my mind was finished. Every single word, every single emotion I felt while a story or conversation was happening in my mind was so realistic and so synched with my emotions. It was like I was doing it in real life.

It was disruptive too and negatively affected the quality of my work and my life in general. I had been late to work and missed deadlines and family gatherings because of my mind's inability to focus.

I struggled to return to reality. I begged my mind, "Don't let them in, don't let them in. Please don't let them in." But my mind won't listen so I talked to the other voices instead. "Go away, please. Go away. Stay away from me." When that didn't work either, I decided to do a different tactic, gripping on words that I had control over. I chanted, "I will not let you in. I will not let you in. I will not let you in. I am walking. I own my mind. I will not let you in."

I straightened up, focused on where I was going, and walked towards the office. A feeling of satisfaction went over me when I saw the office door.

"Yes! I made it. I am here! I'm good. I am really positive about it. This is going to be a very good day." I went in with a smile.

Reflections over coffee is life.

A colleague passed by my cubicle and said, "Coffee?" The magic word that signals it is break time. I stretched my hands upward, leaned back, and stretched my legs.

"I deserve to have my coffee," I told myself. After all, I finished responding to all my emails, made all the pending calls, and submitted a report. "Whew! I am a workhorse!" I imagined patting myself on the back.

I reached for my mug in my lower desk drawer, already imagining the smell and taste of freshly-brewed coffee mixed with my favorite fresh milk, stood up, and walked happily towards the pantry. I went straight to the coffee maker like it's a weapon that must be acquired before going to a battlefield, poured ¾ of my mug with hot coffee, and added some fresh milk.

"This is my type of coffee." I raised my mug a little bit like I was offering a toast (or maybe I need a toast with my coffee), and smiled as I took my first sip of coffee – Arabica or Excelsa? I like both.

I looked for my favorite spot – the high stool just beside the glass window with the view of the city.

I sat on the stool and enjoyed my empowering coffee. The pantry became alive as other colleagues walked in to get their coffee. Woohoo! Fifteen minutes of pure coffee bliss.

"How was the trip up north?" A colleague asked. I traveled last week to close a deal. It was a big one and during these difficult times, a big help to the company.

"Very, very productive," I replied. 'It was one of those times where you thought things would be good and then it ended up being extremely good." We both laughed and sipped our coffee at almost the same time. It was funny and made us laugh even more. I was very, very glad that I worked in this inclusive and collaborative environment, surrounded by colleagues who care about each other. This is not just work, this is family.

I took one more sip of my coffee, closed my eyes, and smiled as I savored its taste and smell. I watched my colleagues in admiration as they talked with each other. I adjusted my seat as I felt that I was starting to lean more on one side. Then, I looked at my colleagues again but something had changed. It was one of those times when you just know instinctively that something happened although nothing did. Well, this was one of those moments. I felt alone, which was stupid. The more that I think about how stupid the feeling was, the lonelier I get. I felt myself retreating into an invisible shell. It's very difficult to explain!

"What are you doing?" I asked myself. "Why are you feeling this stupid feeling?" There was no answer for me and I knew I could not fight it so I just allowed myself to drown in that feeling. Then, I stood up, washed my mug, and told myself, "I am happy being alone."

I went back to my desk and went back to work, convinced that it was my destiny to be a nomad, a passive passerby in each phase of my life. My Instagram account should be "the wanderer" but it's already taken.

I am pretty sure there are other people out there who also feel alone even when in a big group." I told myself.

"Maybe there's a way I can get together with them. We will all be alone together." I shook my head, disapproving of my own stupid thoughts.

I finally gathered enough willpower to refocus my mind on my work.

A good lunch always helps.

Lunch was a tricky part of the day. There were times that one hour was too short, gone before I could finish happy conversations with colleagues. Other times, lunch was too long, going on and on and on. But there were also times when I did not even notice lunch time because my mind was too occupied with its own series of events or my heart was too busy being lonely and then loathing the feeling of being lonely.

On a good day, lunch would be going downstairs and getting takeout food to eat in the pantry or dine-in in a nearby al fresco restaurant with colleagues. I especially loved the group lunch we had two weeks ago at the al fresco restaurant because the vibe was so jolly and positive. There was a happy noise all around. I got to laugh and talk. I talked loudly and was just normal, like everyone else. I ordered pistachio ice cream for dessert and loved it.

A regular, unremarkable day would be having lunch for thirty minutes in the pantry with some conversations, and then returning to my table to nap, which our office calls a power nap, for a few minutes to recharge for the afternoon work. My power nap yesterday was really helpful in ensuring that I had enough energy to last the day without crying.

But on some days, lunchtime also triggers so many emotions in me that it makes continuing with the rest of the day a struggle.

You see, it was supposed to be a happy lunchtime when my father almost killed me when I was 11 years old. I was playing outside with my younger siblings, my mother was working, and my father was cooking lunch. He finished his work early so he was able to cook lunch for us. He cooked wonderful soup with little shrimps in it and excitedly called us to eat lunch.

As soon as we heard my father saying, "Lunch is ready," we forgot the game we were playing and ran towards the house. Toys, leaves, and twigs were scattered as we raced trying to be the first to enter the house. I got to the table first. I was greeted by the inviting sight of shrimps in the soup. We all sat around the table. My father stood up to get a serving spoon. While he was getting the spoon, I looked at the shrimps and they seemed like they were talking to me. "Get one and taste it." I tried to resist but my 11-year-old mind's ability to resist and my hungry stomach's growl were a deadly combination. I leaned and took out a shrimp. Its size was about an inch long.

Unfortunately, at that same moment, my father turned to return to the table and saw me getting the shrimp out of the bowl. I didn't have time to duck as everything happened so fast. He cursed and while cursing, he grabbed me by my throat and told me how horrible and greedy I was. I struggled to breathe as his grip on my neck got stronger and more angry words came out of his mouth. I did not remember the words but I remembered the pain from the hands of a 40-year-old, 80-kilogram man on the throat of a frail 11-year-old girl. My father was big, I was thin and small. I remembered the fear and the disbelief as my eyes grew wide with shock.

When my father's anger subsided, he realized what he had done. He saw that I couldn't breathe and released my neck. In a much softer but still angry voice, he said, "You shouldn't have done that. I cooked that for all of you. Don't be greedy and selfish." At that moment I felt ashamed for what I did. One of my hands was holding my neck, crying, while my other hand was still holding the shrimp. I ate quietly between sobs.

As I grew older, my resentment also grew. What I did was wrong but I was 11 years old, hungry and tempted. That was too much punishment for an 11-year-old. And then there was the question that made me feel alone and unwanted, "Would my father really kill me for a shrimp or was he just so angry at my bad behavior that he snapped and just reacted without thinking?" Then, I would start feeling guilty and blame myself for my father's reaction and my emotional turmoil.

We were poor and to have shrimp for lunch, no matter how small, was a luxury. There was just one shrimp allocated for each family member. Maybe that's why my father snapped. When I took that one shrimp when it was not yet distributed, I also robbed one of my siblings of a chance to get a share. Over the years, I rationalized it. I tried to understand it but the memory never fails to trigger a paralyzing emotional response from me.

There were no physical scars, but every time I remember it the emotional pain would choke me, followed by the opening of a hollow, dark pit in my heart that would swallow my entire being in despair and pity for myself. I loved my father and I appreciated the lengths he went to just to provide for the family, but the spirit of an 11-year-old girl was broken that day and the memory continues to break the spirit of the adult me over and over and over again.

When I have this kind of lunch, when I remember all these sad and bad things, I end up using the rest of my lunch break to wipe my tears away, keep my emotions in check, bring myself back to now, force myself to be ready to get to work again and to not give in to the desire to look for a bed, lie down and cover myself in a blanket while I scream and cry.

Lunchtime was almost over by the time I realized that I had not eaten my food yet. I gobbled my food, almost choking several times, and went back to the office as fast as I could.

Tired using the word tired.

By 2:00pm, I was tired. I was editing a report and was working quite well until I reached a paragraph where my mind automatically rerouted itself to other scenarios and locations. An image of a college friend popped into my mind and I recalled all the happy memories I had with my college friends – watching movies together, singing along with the crowd while watching concerts, getting drunk together to grieve failed exams, and getting into heated debates over national policies while munching chips and drinking soda.

"Oh...how I wish I was back to that age. An age when there was so much hope in my heart. An age when there was so much to look forward to when the world was there for me to discover. An age when I couldn't wait to start changing the world for the better. It was an age when there was that certainty in my heart that after graduation, things would be better and that I could make things better." I was talking to myself again.

"How I miss that feeling, the innocence and the simplicity of things." I sighed with gloom.

"Go away!" I shook my head vigorously, willing away the distracting thoughts.   Once my mind was clear, I went back to work.

"There! You're a genius, Annie! That's what's needed in this report." I triumphantly told myself. All my ideas were coming too fast so I needed to write them down. I took out a pen and paper and quickly wrote down my ideas, my hand trying to keep up with my brain. I wrote really fast but after a few entries, I stopped. My ideas were gone.

"Where did they go?" I read and reread what I've written down, hoping that by doing so I would remember the rest. I looked at my computer screen again and the breaking news popped out of the screen. It was about a politician justifying his association with a recently arrested illegal drugs smuggler. I read it silently, and, in my mind, an alternative event occurred where I was the main character and where I had the power to change the course of the story. I tried to fight the urge to have the story continue in my head but it was so strong.

I stopped working on my laptop and started working on the files on my desk instead. I was hoping the physical movement would disrupt the most recent disruption in my head, but the alternate story was fighting for my headspace, so I gave in. I looked at my files but did nothing. I was busy watching my mind play out the alternate version of the story. I just realized too, that even though the story was in my mind, somehow it was like watching a movie. The scenes were so vivid and the audio was so clear. It felt so weird. "How can I watch something that I cannot see?"

I felt tired and sad and just wanted to go to sleep. My eyes were getting heavy when a sudden surge of energy ran through me. I sat up so quickly, I felt like the upper half of my body got detached and flew up, away from my lower half. It's almost COB! It's going to be close of business soon, which is 5:00PM in our office and I am not yet done looking at this report.

"What is wrong with me? What is wrong with me?" And just like an ever-loyal friend, my mind responded, "A lot…"

I wanted to scream. I was clinching my teeth together so tight; I was afraid my jaw was going to break. I made a silent scream and for a split second everything went blank. My heart was beating so fast I was scared I actually made a sound when I silently screamed.

I had to stay in the office for two more hours to finish editing the report. By the time I finished attaching the file and hitting the send button of the email to send it to my supervisor, I was exhausted, drained, and depressed. If only my mind did not make detours, all I needed were two hours to finish my work. I just wanted to go home, to just be able to sit anywhere in the house, curse, cry and not worry about anyone seeing me and passing judgement.

Will it be home sweet home?

I slowly opened my apartment door, childishly half-expecting to see a magical world, with talking trees, multi-colored birds, and harps floating in the air. I knew it was a crazy thought but I was still disappointed when I was greeted by my worn-out couch and old electric fan.

I was too tired to cook dinner so I opened a canned meatloaf and some old bread. I just realized how hungry I was when I was ready to eat.

"Wow!" That priceless feeling of food touching your mouth when you're tired and hungry. I was halfway through when the thought of staying healthy entered my mind. I looked at the food in front of me and felt guilty and disgusted in equal measure. I felt so guilty for not taking care of my body well and I felt disgusted that I gave in to eating unhealthy food.

"Is there anything in this world that I will ever do right? I asked myself.

I put down my remaining bread and canned meatloaf on the table and stared at it. I started to cry again.

"I hate myself. I hate my life. I hate the world." I said loudly and angrily.

"Is this life worth living?" I blurted out loud but the moment I said it I got scared at the intensity of emotions that came with the question. I was scared of taking the path where answering the question could lead me. "No, please. Not that road." I pleaded with myself.

"Ahhhhh!" I let out a stifled moan.

I looked at my photo on top of the small bookshelf and talked aloud as if confiding to it. "People always say they admire my strength but I can barely hold myself together. My sanity is hanging by a thread and that thread is getting more and more fragile with each passing day.

When people tell me I am strong and brave, I just reply with a smile. What people do not know is that I smile not because I am happy they see me as strong and brave, but because I know that if I say any word at all, I will cry. They have no idea how weak I feel. They have no idea how much I would love to just hug someone and cry. They have no idea how messed up I feel. They have no idea that I am a prisoner of my own mind. I am not free." I stared at the photo intently.

Was my smile in that photo real when it was taken? Was I really happy at that time? I smiled weakly. "You know what? You really are a strong woman. You've been through a lot. You are going through a lot and yet you still manage to be good and kind. Maybe you truly inspire others. Isn't staying alive when you're going through hell strength?" I imagined me in the photo nodding her head.

I reached out for my photo and hugged it. "It's okay to feel weak. You will be strong again. You are amazing and wonderful and you have every right to be in this world. You will find your place again and you will be happy." I hugged my photo tighter.

The warmth from my tears falling down on both sides of my cheeks somehow felt like a warm embrace for my heart. I smiled at the thought that even though I was alone, somehow, I was getting an embrace. Maybe there really is a God and he has not abandoned me. When I was a little girl, I heard someone say that God gives his toughest battles to his strongest soldiers. The thought comforted me. I felt like I was part of a bigger cause and a bigger group of people tasked with a bigger purpose.

I got up from my bed. Stood up and started pacing the floor. I looked outside. It was dark but not that dark as there were street lights. I looked up and stared for a few seconds at the full moon. When you look at the moon quite intently, you can actually see the contours on its face and the variations of gray in its entire circle.

When I was a little girl, the moon was a great source of fascination for me. I spent hours playing with it. Yes, I played with the moon. I used to stand still, look at the moon, and play a staring game with it. Then, I would laugh and run, and behold, the moon would be running after me. I would stop and just walk and the moon would move slowly too. Wherever I went, it followed me without delay. I felt so special in the certainty that the moon was my playmate. I boasted to my friends that I had a special relationship with the moon, my playmate.

"Ahhh.." The sheer delight of playing with the moon. The memory was a priceless treasure.

When I was not in the mood to play, I used to just stare at the moon, look at its gray spots, and think of all the stories about it that my grandmother used to tell me at night. She used to tell me stories about a lazy little boy named Juan who was sent to the moon as a punishment. He was not allowed to return to his family, ever.

My grandmother said that if you look hard enough at the moon, you will see the silhouette of a boy riding a carabao who was sent to the moon as a punishment because he was extremely lazy. Another story was that of the doomed lovers who chose to be banished to the moon to stay together. I used to look at the moon and wonder which silhouette would be shown first – that of Juan and his carabao or the faces of the doomed sweethearts looking at each other.

The first time I read about the moon landing, I started seeing myself walking on the moon. I wanted to be an astronaut, go to the moon, and meet Juan and his carabao. I even thought that maybe I could take Juan and his carabao home with me. I was so sure he would be glad to be back on Earth.

Those younger years were the happy, carefree days. I loved those days. I live for the memories of those days. I live for moments like these when my heart is full of gratitude and happiness. I looked at the moon again. Thank you moon. I smiled, closed my eyes, clasped my hands together on my lap, and prayed. After praying, I prepared to have a good night's sleep.

Tomorrow will be better. I know what I will do tomorrow.

Seeing hope amidst the pockets of pain.

The next morning, I prepared early, confident of what I needed to do. What I realized last night was I did not have to and I could not do this on my own anymore. My mind and I needed help.

I told my mind, "I still have many, many years ahead of me and I want to live a life where I can be present in the NOW, to actually live right in the moment, and to not escape in another world that existed only in my mind. I need to face my ghosts, open my pain pockets, and deal with them one by one.

I understand that my life will not change overnight but I would like to take the small steps in making my life better. I need to take care of myself so I can also take care of my loved ones and nurture the beautiful relationships that I have with my friends and family. I need to be better. My heart needs to heal. My mind needs to be healthy." My mind agreed with me.

I got off the bus and stood at the gate of the psychologist's office. It was made of metal and old wood. The wooden part looked like it was designed based on the imperfections of the log –

and the imperfections made it look perfect. I tentatively pressed the doorbell, not sure if I wanted someone to open the gate and let me in or for the gate to remain closed so I could go home while telling myself, "It was not meant to be. At least I tried." As my mind debated the best scenario for me, the gate opened. I was greeted by a welcoming, beautiful garden, with lots of flowering plants with different colors and a round garden table with four chairs.

There was a small pathway on the side of the flowering plants that led to a sunroom. We entered the sunroom, walked past potted plants, and entered another door. The room was more subdued, with only one potted green plant with leaves that looked like small coconut palm leaves. The plant was on the corner opposite the door.

It is a relatively small room, maybe 20 square meters in area. On one side, there was a rug with three square pillows on it. On the other side, there was a couch that could seat two people opposite a couch for just one occupant. We walked towards the couches. The psychologist asked me to sit wherever I felt most comfortable. I chose to sit on the single-occupant couch. The psychologist then sat on the opposite couch.

"Are you comfortable?"

"Yes", I replied.

I was asked if I wanted water or coffee. I declined both. I was not in the mood to drink or eat anything. I was eager, nervous, scared, and excited all at the same time. I took a deep breath and smiled. The psychologist started talking. She was saying all these nice things. I think she was trying to make me feel welcome and was trying to establish rapport with me. I read somewhere that that's what psychologists do first. I listened attentively.

"This is a safe space. My approach is I will wait for you until you are ready to share, to talk, to engage. If you just want to sit here and reflect or just relax or just to have a quiet space for yourself, you can do it here." I nodded my head, smiled weakly, and took a deep breath again.

"So, I don't have to say anything unless I am ready to do so," I quietly told my mind. That was reassuring. I looked at the psychologist. There was no expression on the face but it looked friendly and not threatening. The effect it had on me was to panic a little bit. The silence while in the room with another person, someone I was seeing for the first time was unsettling. Strangely, though, I also felt calm and my mind was not doing its usual storytelling. I just didn't know where to start.

I looked at the plant. I looked at the candles, which I assumed were scented, carefully arranged on the small coffee table beside the potted plant. I leaned back and rested my back and head on the couch. Then, I closed my eyes.

The first thing I noticed was the tear coming out of my right eye. Well, actually, I did not notice the tears. What I noticed was my reaction. My hand went up to my eye with the back of my palm wiping away the tears. As soon as I realized tears were falling from my right eye, tears from the left eye followed, and more tears came, and from the quiet falling of tears, a sob escaped from my throat, followed by a soft cry. And then, my eyes unleashed a flash flood of tears. I cried uncontrollably, with my shoulders shaking and my heart racing.

I was rocking back and forth with both my hands on my mouth. Maybe I was trying to stifle the crying sound, or maybe I was trying to make myself stop, or maybe I was using my hands to support myself. I did not really know. When I calmed down, I started talking, slowly at first.

"I came here because I think I need help. There were so many things that happened in my life. I thought I was on top of everything. I thought I would be okay. But I am not okay and I fear that I am going to reach my breaking point really, really soon." That was all I could say before I started sobbing again.

It was difficult to survive one pain after another without breaking down so to survive I developed an internal system where I wrapped the pain in an imaginary single pocket and put it in a tightly locked storage inside my heart. The pocket was thick and could be completely zipped so the pain could not easily come out unless I allowed it.

I was an expert in compartmentalizing and hiding the pain. However, as time passed by, the pockets of pain became too many and my heart too heavy. It was difficult to carry all those pockets of pain year after year after year. I didn't know where to store the new ones anymore. Time wore down the existing pockets and loosened the zippers threatening to spill the pain in each pocket on the slightest emotional trigger. The burden of too many pockets and worn-out pockets was wearing me down and destroying my mental health. I needed to unload.

I mentally chose the first pocket that I was ready to open. I carefully allowed my heart to let go of the pocket and emptied its pain. I imagined unzipping the pocket and started talking. I talked more and more and more. I cried more too.

After the session, the room looked a little brighter, the plants were more vibrant, and the people walking on the street were a little nicer. Everything around me just felt a little lighter. Of course, I could not say yet if my life will be better in the long run but I am glad that I decided to do this.

I would trade anything in this world right now for this feeling of lightness knowing that there's a little bit more space in my heart for hope. And I will keep on working to make that space bigger so hope would live permanently in my heart. I smiled and thanked God. Then, I looked again at the people around me, all strangers, and sent a silent request, which I hope would reach their hearts, "Please pray for me. I pray for you too."

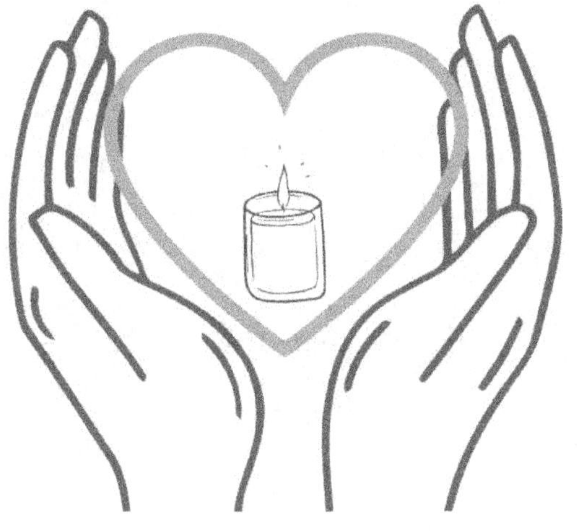